ICS 11.202

SCM

世界中医药学会联合会
World Federation of Chinese Medicine Societies

SCM 0051-2019

国际中医远程会诊服务规范

Specifications for International Chinese Medicine Telemedicine Service

世界中联国际组织标准
International Standard of WFCMS

2019-12-26发布实施
Issued & implemented on December 26th, 2019

中医古籍出版社
Publishing House of Ancient Chinese Medical Books

图书在版编目（CIP）数据

国际中医远程会诊服务规范：汉英对照 / 世界中医药学会联合会著 . —北京：中医古籍出版社，2020.7
ISBN 978-7-5152-2141-0

Ⅰ . ①国… Ⅱ . ①世… Ⅲ . ①中医学—远程会诊—医疗卫生服务—规范—汉、英 Ⅳ . ① R44-65

中国版本图书馆 CIP 数据核字（2020）第 097881 号

国际中医远程会诊服务规范
世界中医药学会联合会　著

责任编辑　王晓曼
出版发行　中医古籍出版社
社　　址　北京东直门内南小街 16 号（100700）
电　　话　010-64089446（总编室）010-64002949（发行部）
网　　址　www.zhongyiguji.com.cn
印　　刷　北京建宏印刷有限公司
开　　本　880mm×1230mm　1/16
印　　张　1.5
字　　数　45 千字
版　　次　2020 年 7 月第 1 版　2020 年 7 月第 1 次印刷
书　　号　ISBN 978-7-5152-2141-0
定　　价　36.00 元

目　　次

前　　言

本标准主要起草单位：

中　　国：江苏省中医院（南京中医药大学附属医院）

本标准参与起草单位：

美　　国：洛杉矶中医药大学

加 拿 大：加拿大多伦多华助中心

英　　国：英国兰维多利亚学院

澳大利亚：澳大利亚红卫连锁中医诊所

瑞　　士：瑞士 TCMENERGIE 健康科技投资集团

荷　　兰：荷兰江苏商会、欧洲传统医药科学学院

智　　利：智利华助中心、智利中医药协会

本标准主要起草人：

中　　国：方祝元、束雅春、宁丽琴、史海波、陈列红、寇建秋、邹建东、黄芳

本标准参与起草人：

美　　国：黎洪

加 拿 大：倪张俊

英　　国：汤淑兰

澳大利亚：沈红卫

瑞　　士：章凌云、Ms. Michelle

荷　　兰：胡绮、王维祥、陈琳

智　　利：王何兴、杨剑波

本标准的起草程序遵守了世界中医药学会联合会发布的 SCM 0001–2009《标准制定和发布工作规范》和 2019 年发布的《世界中医药学会联合会国际组织标准管理办法》。

国际中医远程会诊服务规范

1 范围

本文件规定了开展国际中医远程会诊服务的机构组织形式、基本条件、工作流程以及管理要求等方面内容。

本文件适用于国际中医远程会诊服务的实施与管理。

2 规范性引用文件

下列文件对于本文件的应用必不可少。凡是标注日期的引用文件，仅标注日期的版本适用于本文件。凡是不标注日期的引用文件，其最新版本（包括所有的修改单）适用于本文件。

WS/T529–2016 远程医疗信息系统基本功能规范

WS/T545–2017 远程医疗信息系统技术规范

WS/T546–2017 远程医疗信息系统与统一通信平台交互规范

SCM 0002–2007 中医基本名词术语中英对照国际标准

3 术语和定义

下列术语和定义适用于本文件。

3.1 国际中医远程会诊

两个或两个以上国家或地区医疗机构之间利用通讯、计算机及网络技术，采用离线或在线交互方式，开展远程中医诊疗指导、协助远程中医诊断、出具诊断意见和远程会诊报告等中医会诊服务活动的过程。

3.2 邀请方

在国际中医远程会诊服务中，发起远程会诊需求的医疗机构或该医疗机构的代理机构。

3.3 受邀方

在国际中医远程会诊服务中，根据邀请方发起的会诊需求，提供远程会诊服务的医疗机构或该医疗机构的代理机构。

3.4 患者

在国际中医远程会诊服务中，患某种疾病并接受会诊服务的人。

3.5 国际中医远程诊断

在国际中医远程会诊服务中，邀请方向受邀方提出申请并提供患者临床资料，受邀方根据患者资料，通过线上望、闻、问等诊断方法，结合邀请方切脉所获得的数据进行综合分析，出具中医诊断意见的过程。

3.6 国际中医远程会诊服务平台

两个国家或地区医疗机构或其代理机构之间运用通讯、计算机及网络技术等信息化手段，为患者提供中医会诊服务的远程平台。

4 组织形式

4.1 通过已搭建的国际中医远程会诊服务平台，邀请方、受邀方以机构身份在该平台注册。

4.2 邀请方通过该平台发布中医会诊需求，由国际中医远程会诊服务平台匹配受邀方或其他中医医疗机构，对需求作出应答，为患者提供中医远程会诊服务。

4.3 邀请方、受邀方通过协议明确责、权、利。

5 基本条件

5.1 机构

5.1.1 开展国际中医远程会诊的机构应在所在国家或地区具有合法的执业资质。

5.1.2 开展国际中医远程会诊机构的远程会诊行为必须符合所在国家或地区的法律、法规。

5.1.3 开展国际中医远程会诊的机构均应有在本机构注册、符合国际中医远程会诊服务要求的中医专业技术人员。

5.1.4 开展国际中医远程会诊的机构应具有相应的国际中医远程会诊服务管理制度，以及医疗质量、医疗安全、信息化技术保障措施。

5.2 人员

5.2.1 中医执业人员

邀请方与受邀方应当根据患者病情安排相应级别的中医师参与国际中医远程会诊服务。邀请方至少有 1 名执业中医师陪同；受邀方至少有 1 名具有相应中医诊疗服务能力、独立开展中医临床工作至少 3 年以上的执业中医师为患者提供中医远程会诊服务。

5.2.2 信息技术人员

远程会诊医疗机构内需有专职人员负责仪器、远程设备、信息系统等设施的定期检测、登记、维护、改造等，符合中医远程会诊相关信息标准和信息安全的规定，保障远程会诊服务信息系统（硬件和软件）处于正常运行状态。

5.2.3 翻译人员

在国际中医远程会诊服务中，若邀请方与受邀方语言不同，需有一方配备 1 名熟练掌握相应语种的翻译人员。

5.3 设备设施

5.3.1 国际中医远程会诊信息系统应当满足图像、声音、文字以及中医诊疗所需要求，确保信息安全、实时传输、图像清晰、数据准确，符合相关国家或地区远程会诊信息系统建设要求，满足中医远程会诊要求。

5.3.2 重要设备和网络应当配备不间断电源。

5.3.3 国际中医远程会诊服务网络需保持稳定、畅通，保障远程会诊服务信息顺利传输。有条件的邀请方、受邀方可以建设国际中医远程医疗专网。

6 工作流程

6.1 签订合作协议

邀请方和受邀方需签订国际中医远程会诊合作协议，约定合作目的、合作条件、合作内容、远程会诊流程、各方责权利、损害风险等事项。

注：合作协议可以签订电子文件。

6.2 知情同意

邀请方应当根据患者的病情和意愿，组织国际中医远程会诊服务，向患者说明远程会诊服务的内容、费用等情况，并征得患者同意；不宜向患者说明病情的，应当征得其监护人或者近亲属同意。双方根据不同情形，签订相关协议。

6.3 发出邀请

邀请方提出邀请，邀请内容至少应包括邀请事由、目的、时间安排、患者相关病历摘要及拟邀请中医师的专业和技术职务、任职资格等。

6.4 接受邀请

受邀方接到邀请方发出的国际中医远程会诊服务邀请后，要及时作出是否接受邀请的决定。若接受邀请，须告知邀请方，并做好相关准备工作；若不接受邀请，应及时告知邀请方并说明理由。

6.5 实施服务

——邀请方和受邀方形成两个国家或地区医疗机构之间的合作关系。

——由邀请方收集患者临床资料，受邀方接受邀请后，应及时并认真负责地安排具备相应资质和技术能力的中医师，按照相关法律、法规等要求，提供国际中医远程会诊服务，及时将会诊意见告知邀请方，并出具由会诊医师签名的会诊意见报告。

——邀请方根据患者临床资料，结合双方望、闻、问、切等诊断方法所获得的数据综合分析，参考受邀方的会诊意见，确定中医诊断与治疗方案。

——根据患者病情，可提供中医远程多学科联合会诊服务。

6.6 资料保存

邀请方、受邀方应按照相应国家或地区病历书写及保管的有关规定共同完成病历资料的填写工作，原件一式两份，由邀请方、受邀方分别归档保存。中医远程会诊服务相关文书可通过电子文件等方式发送。若双方医务人员仅为患者提供咨询服务，也应及时记录信息。

7 管理要求

7.1 机构管理

7.1.1 制定并落实管理规章制度，参与远程会诊的医疗机构需执行所在国家或地区发布或者认可的中医远程诊疗技术规范和操作规程，在双方法律框架下保障医疗质量与安全。

7.1.2 开展国际中医远程会诊服务的医疗机构应设置专门的医疗质量安全管理部门或配备专职人员，负责国际中医远程会诊服务质量管理与控制工作。

7.1.3 医疗质量安全管理人员应当具备相关专业知识和工作经验。

7.1.4 作为邀请方、受邀方的代理机构，应与邀请方、受邀方签订相关协议，通过协议明确各方权利、义务和法律责任，落实财务管理等各项制度。

7.2 人员管理

7.2.1 制定并落实相关医务人员、信息技术人员、支持服务人员的培训计划，保证其具备相关的专业知识与服务能力。

7.2.2 在提供中医远程会诊服务时，应当遵守所有参与方国家或地区的医疗、药品管理等相关法律、法规，并按照合作协议约定的内容提供服务，履行相关义务，承担相应责任。

7.3 质量管理

7.3.1 依据所在国家或地区法律、法规，实行患者实名制管理，建立相关管理制度、人员岗位职责、服务流程等国际中医远程会诊服务管理体系。

7.3.2 督促落实各项规章制度和日常远程医疗管理工作，并对中医远程会诊服务行为进行监督和检查。

7.3.3 规范使用和管理远程会诊设备、信息系统设备，对中医远程会诊设备、信息系统进行日常维护，保证其正常运转。

7.3.4 建立良好的医患沟通机制，维护患者合法权益。

7.4 费用管理

7.4.1 建立国际中医远程会诊服务的财务管理制度。

7.4.2　邀请方、受邀方达成一致并签订的协议中，关于费用主要包括：

——全部费用及明细；

——支付方式；

——支付出现问题时的解决措施。

7.4.3　受邀方应为邀请方提供多种支付方式，当选用某种支付方式将产生额外费用时，应在支付前向邀请方的医疗机构说明。

7.4.4　在支付完成后，受邀方应向邀请方提供支付凭证。

注：在双方或多方达成一致的情况下，根据各方条件，可以选择电汇、转账、微信、支付宝等支付方式。

7.5　安全管理

参与国际中医远程会诊的各方应当加强信息安全和患者隐私保护，防止违法传输、修改，防止数据丢失，建立数据安全管理规程，确保网络安全、操作安全、数据安全和隐私安全。

8　争议及纠纷处理

医疗机构之间或医疗机构与代理机构之间合作开展国际中医远程会诊服务发生争议或纠纷时，按照相关法律、法规和双方或多方已达成的合作协议约定内容进行处理，并承担相应责任。

9　服务评价与改进

9.1　建立服务评价管理机制，定期接受服务评价。

9.2　服务评价活动应符合如下基本要求：

——具备科学的评价方案，评价行为依据评价方案开展；

——采集使用真实的数据，评价结果客观准确地反映评价对象真实情况，具有高信度；

——评价内容与实际工作一致，具有高效度。

9.3　评价者根据不同评价目标，从规范性附录 A 中根据实际情况，选取合适的评价指标并进行细化、组合、赋权，实施具体评价活动。

9.4　服务提供者根据服务评价结果，制定整改措施，持续改进，不断提高服务水平。

附录 A

（规范性附录）

国际中医远程会诊服务评价指标

表 A.1 国际中医远程会诊服务评价指标

序号	一级指标	二级指标
1	医疗机构基本条件	开展国际中医远程会诊服务的医疗机构应当具有相应执业资质
2		医疗机构或其代理机构必须在本国的法律范围内，被允许开展国际中医远程会诊服务，远程会诊行为必须符合所在国家或地区的法律、法规
3		双方医疗机构均有在本机构注册、符合中医远程会诊服务要求的中医专业技术人员
4		远程会诊服务机构具有医疗质量与医疗安全、信息化技术保障措施
5	医师基本条件	参与中医远程会诊的双方医师均有执业中医师资质
6		受邀方医疗机构安排独立开展临床工作至少 3 年以上的执业中医师开展远程会诊服务
7	支持人员基本条件	医疗机构内需有专职人员负责仪器、远程设备、设施的定期检测、登记、维护等
8		医疗机构有专人负责远程医疗信息系统的调试与维护
9		医疗机构配有专为中医远程会诊服务提供咨询、联系沟通等服务的专业人员
10	设备设施基本条件	国际中医远程会诊信息系统应当满足图像、声音、文字以及中医诊疗所需要求
11		远程会诊服务网络应确保系统稳定、畅通
12		重要设备和网络应当配备不间断电源
13	远程会诊工作流程	参与国际远程会诊服务的机构已签订中医远程会诊合作协议
14		中医远程会诊服务合作协议内容全面
15		邀请方根据患者病情和意愿，组织国际中医远程会诊服务，并向患者说明远程会诊服务内容、费用等情况，征得患者同意
16		不宜向患者说明病情的，应当征得其监护人或者近亲属同意，并签订相关协议
17		医疗机构有邀请方提供的远程会诊服务申请（可为纸质版或电子版）
18		受邀方安排的远程会诊服务中医师，具备相应资质和技术能力，符合要求
19		参与国际中医远程会诊服务的医疗机构有相关医师签名的诊疗意见或会诊报告
20		中医远程会诊服务中相关会诊文件书写符合规范
21		参与国际中医远程会诊服务的医疗机构将患者的相关远程会诊病历资料存档、保管符合要求

序号	一级指标	二级指标
22	机构人员质量管理要求	国际中医远程会诊服务机构各项规章制度健全，并落实到位
23		远程会诊服务人员能按中医诊疗常规、技术规范、操作规程等进行远程会诊服务
24		对影响医疗质量及安全的高危因素有防范措施
25		远程会诊服务机构具有防止医疗数据、患者信息泄露及数据丢失等安全措施
26		与代理机构合作开展中医远程会诊服务者，各方责、权、利明确
27		双方或多方医疗机构及医务人员遵守所在国家或地区的相关法律法规，执行相关技术规范和标准
28		远程会诊服务机构实行患者实名制管理
29		医疗质量安全管理人员能定期对远程会诊服务质量、制度落实等进行检查，有记录
30		建立医患沟通机制
31		规范使用和管理远程会诊设备、信息系统设备
32	费用管理	国际中医远程会诊服务机构有财务管理制度，并落实
33		参与远程会诊服务机构双方签订的协议中包含费用明细、支付方式
34		远程会诊服务机构对于远程会诊完成支付者能提供支付凭证
35	安全管理	参与国际中医远程会诊的各方应有确保网络安全、操作安全、数据安全、保护患者隐私的制度与防范措施
36		参与国际中医远程会诊的各方应当建立数据安全管理规程，保护患者隐私，防止违法传输、修改，防止数据丢失
37	争议处理	远程会诊服务机构各方均有争议或纠纷处理约定，并符合各国法律规定
38	服务评价与改进	中医远程会诊服务提供机构有针对国际中医远程会诊服务的评价管理机制，并能实施具体评价活动，评价方案科学、可操作
39		采集数据真实，评价结果客观、准确，具有高信度
40		中医远程会诊服务提供机构能根据评价结果，就存在问题制定整改措施，持续改进，有记录

Foreword

Main drafting organization: Jiangsu Provincial Hospital of Chinese Traditional Medicine (Affiliated Hospital of Nanjing University of Chinese Traditional Medicine)

Drafting organizations participated:
US: Los Angeles TCM University
Canada: Toronto Overseas Chinese Service Center
UK: Shulan College of Chinese UK
Australia: Hongwei TCM Chain Clinic
Switzerland: TCM Energie Health Technology Investment Group
Holland: Dutch Chamber of Commerce (Jiangsu), European Academy of Traditional Medical Science
Chile: Overseas Chinese Service Center, Chile TCM Association

Main drafters:
China: Fang Zhuyuan, Shu Yachun, Ning Liqin, Shi Haibo, Chen Liehong, Kou Jianqiu, Zou Jiandong, Huang Fang

Drafters participated:
US: Li Hong
Canada: Ni Zhangjun
UK: Tang Shulan
Australia: Shen Hongwei
Switzerland: Zhang Lingyun, Ms.Michelle
Holland: Hu Qi, Wang Weixiang, Chen Lin
Chile: Wang Hexing, Yang Jianbo

The drafting procedures of this Standard conform to the SCM 0001-2009 Specifications on Standard Formulation and Publishing issued by World Federation of Chinese Medicine Societies and Regulations on International Standards of WFCMS issued in 2019.

Specifications for International Chinese medicine telemedicine service

1 Scope

This standard specifies the requirements for international Chinese Medicine telemedicine service in terms of organizational forms, basic conditions, processes and management.

This standard is applicable to the implementation and management of the Service.

2 Normative References

The following documents are referred to in the text in such a way that some or all of their content constitutes requirements of this document. For dated references, only the edition cited applies. For undated references, the latest edition of the referenced document (including any amendments) applies.

WS/T529-2016 Specifications for Basic Functions of Telemedicine Information Systems

WS/T545-2017 Technical Specifications for Telemedicine Information Systems

WS/T546-2017 Specifications for Interactions Between Telemedicine Information Systems and Unified Communication Platforms

SCM 0002-2007 International Standard Chinese-English Basic Nomenclature of Chinese Medicine

3 Terms and Definitions

For the purposes of this document, the following terms and definitions apply.

3.1 International Chinese medicine telemedicine service

A process that medical institutions in two or more than two different countries or regions offering remote Chinese Medicine treatment guidance, helping remote Chinese Medicine diagnoses, providing diagnosis-based opinions and issue telemedicine reports and other Chinese Medicine consultation services, on line or off line, by leveraging communication, computer and network techniques.

3.2 Inviter

An institution or an agency which posts a demand for telemedicine in an international Chinese medicine service.

3.3 Invitee

An institution or an agency which provides opinions for the inviter who posts a demand for consultation.

3.4 Patient

A person who suffers from a certain disease and receives consultation service in an international Chinese medicine telemedicine.

3.5 International Chinese medicine remote diagnosis

In an international Chinese medicine telemedicine service, the inviter applies to the invitee and provides a patient's clinical information. The invitee conducts comprehensive Chinese medicine diagnosis through on-line inspection, listening and questioning based on the patient's clinical information, as well as the data the inviting institution has gained through pulse-taking, so as to provide diagnosis-based opinions.

3.6 International Chinese medicine telemedicine service platform

A remote platform that supplies remote Chinese medicine consultation service to patients provided by medical institutions or agencies in two or more than two different countries or regions with communication techniques, computer, internet, etc.

4 Organizational forms

4.1 The invitee and the inviter shall register as an institution on the pre-established international Chinese medicine telemedicine service platform.

4.2 When the inviter posts a demand for Chinese medicine treatment on the platform, the platform will match the invitee or an alternative Chinese medicine institution, as a way to respond to the demand.

4.3 The inviter and invitee involved shall sign an agreement to make clear their respective rights and obligations.

5 Basic Conditions

5.1 Institutions

5.1.1 An institution engaged in the Chinese medicine telemedicine service shall have the qualifications legally required in the country or region.

5.1.2 A medical institution engaged in the Chinese medicine telemedicine service shall abide by the corresponding laws and regulations required in the country or region.

5.1.3 The institutions that carry out the international remote Chinese medicine telemedicine service shall have professional Chinese medicine personnel registered in the institution and meeting the relevant requirements.

5.1.4 The institutions engaged in the Chinese medicine telemedicine service shall establish management systems, medical quality assurance measures, medical safety assurance measures and information-based technical support measures.

5.2 Service personnel

5.2.1 Chinese medicine practitioners

In light of the patient's conditions, the inviter and the invitee shall assign Chinese medicine physicians of appropriate levels to participate in the service. To be precise, the inviter shall assign at least one Chinese medicine practitioner, and the invitee shall assign at least one Chinese medicine practitioner who is competent in Chinese medicine diagnosis and treatment and has at least three years of experience in clinical Chinese medicine service.

5.2.2 Remote consultation service supporters

Medical institutions engaged in telemedicine shall specially assign persons to regularly inspect, register, maintain and renovate instruments, remote equipment, facilities and information systems in ways that follow the information standards and information security provisions applicable to Chinese medicine telemedicine. By doing so, their telemedicine service information systems (hardware and software) shall be kept in a good state that meets demands in Chinese medicine telemedicine.

5.2.3 Translators and interpreters

In the international Chinese medicine remote consultation service, if the languages are different between the inviter and the invitee, one party must be equipped with a translator or interpreter proficient in the corresponding languages.

5.3 Equipment and facilities

5.3.1 An international Chinese medicine remote consultation information system shall meet requirements for image, voice, text and Chinese Medicine diagnosis and treatment, and transmit information securely in real time. Furthermore, clear images and accurate data shall be delivered in ways that fulfill local requirements for telemedicine information systems, as well as demands in Chinese medicine remote clinical diagnosis and treatment.

5.3.2 Major equipment and networks shall be UPS-backed.

5.3.3 An international Chinese medicine telemedicine network shall remain stable and unblocked in the country or region it is located in, and enable telemedicine information to be transmitted seamlessly. If possible, the inviter or invitee may develop a specialized network for international Chinese medicine telemedicine.

6 Working Process

6.1 Signing cooperation agreement

The inviter and invitee shall sign a cooperation agreement for Chinese medicine remote consultation to define the purpose, conditions and content of cooperation, the procedures of telemedicine, the rights and obligations of the parties involved, and the medical damage risks and responsibilities.

Note: Such agreement may be signed electronically.

6.2 Informed consent

The inviter shall organize the service in consideration of the patient's conditions and willingness, explain to the patient details of the service, such as content and costs, and obtain the consent from the patient. In the event that it is inappropriate to disclose to the patient his conditions, an informed consent shall be obtained from his guardian or close relatives. Both sides sign relevant agreement on the basis of specific situations.

6.3 Sending an invitation

The inviter make an invitation to the invitee and the invitation shall encompass the origin and purpose, the schedule, an abstract of the patient's record and expected majors, technical titles and qualifications of invited Chinese medicine physicians.

6.4 Invitation acceptance

When receiving an invitation on the service from the inviter, the invitee shall promptly decide whether to accept the invitation. To accept the invitation entails notifying the inviter and making required preparations. If the invitee decides not to accept the invitation, the invitee shall promptly notify and make an explanation to the inviter.

6.5 Service delivery

—The inviter and the invitee in two countries or regions form a cooperative relationship.

—The invitee shall meticulously assign Chinese medicine physicians with required qualifications and technical competence, and deliver the service in alignment with applicable laws, regulations and specifications for diagnosis and treatment, with diagnosis and treatment opinions timely made known to the inviter. This process shall end with a consultation report signed by the physicians involved.

—The inviter shall develop a Chinese medicine diagnosis and treatment schedule based on the patient's clinical information, comprehensive analysis of the data acquired by the two parties through looking, listening, questioning and pulse taking, as well as the invitee's diagnosis and treatment opinions.

—The remote Chinese medicine multi-disciplinary treatment service may be made available in alignment with the patient's conditions.

6.6 Archive

The inviter and the invitee shall work together to complete medical records in accordance with their local provisions on writing and taking care of medical records. Both the inviter and the invitee shall archive originals of medical records in duplicate. Documents on the service may be sent electronically. In the event that the two parties only deliver a consulting service to the patient, consulting information shall be promptly recorded.

7 Management Requirements

7.1 Institution management

7.1.1 Rules and regulations for the administration of the service shall be developed and put in place. Two medical institutions in different countries shall follow through on technical and operation specifications for Chinese medicine telemedicine issued or approved by their countries or regions, as an approach to medical quality and safety assurance under their countries' legal frameworks.

7.1.2 A medical institution engaged in the service shall specially set up a medical quality and safety management department or assign persons to quality management and control in the service.

7.1.3 Medical quality and safety control managers shall have required expertise and work experience.

7.1.4 As an agency, the institution shall sign an agreement with the inviter and invitee to make clear rights, obligations and legal liabilities of all the parties involved. In addition, various applicable regulations, including those on financial management, shall be put in place.

7.2 Personnel management

7.2.1 Develop and implement training programs for medical personnel, IT technicians and supporters involved in the service, to enable the personnel to gain expertise and competence required by their posts.

7.2.2 When participating in international Chinese medicine telemedicine service shall abide by laws and regulations on remote medical consultation service and drug control of all stakeholder countries while delivering the service, and work in alignment with the service content and fulfill the obligations and responsibilities under the cooperation agreement.

7.3 Quality management

7.3.1 Establish a real-name system for patients and develop relevant management systems, during the international Chinese medicine telemedicine service, including post responsibility, service flow and other systems, according to the laws and regulations of the local country or region

7.3.2 Implement the management rules and regulations and daily telemedicine management work, and supervise and inspect the medical remote consultation service.

7.3.3 Standardize the use and management of remote consultation equipment and information system equipment and have routine maintenance to ensure its normal operation.

7.3.4 Establish a good communication mechanism between doctors and patients to protect the legitimate rights and interests of patients.

7.4 Cost management

7.4.1 A financial management system shall be developed for the service.

7.4.2 The inviter and the invitee shall reach a consensus and sign an agreement that covers:

—all costs and their breakdown;

—modes of payment;

—actions to be taken in the event that a payment fails.

7.4.3 The invitee shall make available multiple payment options to the inviter. When a certain mode of payment incurs additional costs, an explanation shall be made to the inviter before the payment.

7.4.4 When a payment is made, the invitee shall issue a payment voucher to the inviter.

Note: On the premise of consensus, the inviter may opt to pay by telegraphic transfer, transfer, WeChat or Alipay amongst others, subject to conditions of the parties involved.

7.5 Security management

All parties involved in international Chinese medicine telemedicine shall strengthen information security and privacy protection for the patients to prevent illegal transmission, revision and data loss. Data security management specifications should be launched to ensure internet, operation, data and privacy security.

8 Dispute Settlement

In the event that a dispute arises out of the telemedicine service between two medical institutions in different countries, the inviter and the invitee shall settle the dispute under the applicable laws and regulations and the agreement concluded by the two sides and take corresponding responsibility.

9 Evaluation and Improvement

9.1 Develop an evaluation management mechanism, and regularly assess the service.

9.2 The basic requirements of service evaluation shall include:

—be equipped with and follow a scientific assessment scheme;

—collect real data, and reflect how the service proceeds, objectively, accurately and credibly, and;

—align what is assessed to practical work, and be conducted efficiently.

9.3 In light of evaluation objectives, an assessor shall select proper evaluation indicators from the Appendix A, and refine, combine and weight them, for specific evaluation activities according to the prescriptions in Appendix A or specific situations.

9.4 A medical institution engaged in the service shall develop improvement measures, and keep improving the service.

Appendix A

(Normative)

International Chinese Medicine Telemedicine Service Evaluation Index

The evaluation index of international Chinese medicine telemedicine service is shown in the following table A.1.

Table A.1

No.	Primary indicator	Secondary indicator
1	Basic conditions of medical institution	A medical institution engaged in the service shall have required qualifications.
2		To the extent permitted by law, a medical institution engaged in the service must obtain permission to deliver the service in the country it operates in. What it does in the course of the service must abide by laws and regulations of the country it operates in.
3		Either party engaged in the service shall have Chinese medicine technicians who have registered with the party and meet the requirements for the service.
4		A medical institution engaged in the service shall maintain medical quality assurance measures, medical safety assurance measures and information-based technical support measures for the service.
5	Basic conditions of physicians	Either party's physicians involved in the service shall have the Chinese medicine practitioner qualification.
6		The inviter shall assign Chinese medicine practitioners who have at least three years of experience in clinical Chinese medicine service, to the service.
7	Basic conditions of supporters	A medical institution engaged in the service shall specially assign persons to regularly inspect, register and maintain instruments, remote equipment and facilities.
8		A medical institution engaged in the service shall specially assign persons to debug and maintain telemedicine information systems.
9		Professionals engaged in consultation and communication shall be allocated for the service.
10	Basic conditions of equipment and facilities	An international Chinese medicine telemedicine information system shall meet requirements for image, voice, text and Chinese medicine diagnosis and treatment.

No.	Primary indicator	Secondary indicator
11		An international Chinese medicine telemedicine network shall remain stable and unblocked.
12		Major equipment and networks shall be UPS-backed.
13	Telemedicine working process	Institutions involved in the service shall sign a Chinese medicine telemedicine cooperation agreement.
14		The agreement shall be comprehensive.
15		The inviter shall arrange the international Chinese medicine telemedicine service in line with the conditions and willingness of the patient, explain to him about the telemedicine service including its content and cost and obtain the consent of the patient.
16		In the event that it is inappropriate to disclose to a patient his conditions, consent shall be obtained from his guardian or close relatives before relevant agreement is signed.
17		The inviter shall make a telemedicine service application, in printed or electronic form.
18		The invitee's Chinese medicine physicians involved in the service shall have required qualifications and technical competence, and meet applicable requirements.
19		A medical institution engaged in the service shall give a diagnosis and treatment opinion report or consultation report signed by the physicians involved.
20		Medical documents generated in the course of the service shall be standardized.
21		A medical institution engaged in the service shall archive and take good care of patient records related to telemedicine.
22	Management requirements for institution staff quality	A medical institution engaged in the service shall maintain and put in place well-developed rules and regulations.
23		Remote consultation service staff shall work in alignment with common practices and technical and operating specifications of Chinese medicine diagnosis and treatment.
24		Preventive measures shall be developed to address high-risk factors that may undermine medical quality and safety.

No.	Primary indicator	Secondary indicator
25		A medical institution engaged in the service shall maintain measures that prevent disclosures or losses of medical data and patient information.
26		In the event that an agency is involved in the service, responsibilities and rights shall be made clear for all the parties involved.
27		Parties to the service and their medical staff shall abide by laws and regulations of the countries or the regions they operate in, and put in place applicable technical specifications and standards.
28		The medical institution engaged in the service shall put in place a real-name system for patients.
29		Medical quality and safety managers shall regularly inspect the quality of the service and how applicable systems work, with records kept.
30		An effective doctor-patient communication mechanism shall be developed to protect patients' right to informed consent.
31		The operation and control of telemedicine equipment and IT system equipment shall be standardized.
32	Cost management	A medical institution engaged in the service shall develop a financial management system for the service.
33		The agreement concluded by the parties to the service shall cover cost breakdown and modes of payment available.
34		A medical institution engaged in the service shall issue a payment voucher when a payment is made for the service.
35	Security management	All parties involved in international Chinese medicine telemedicine shall put in place institutions and preventive measures that ensure internet, operation and data security and protect the privacy of patients.
36		All parties involved in international Chinese medicine telemedicine shall put in place data security management specifications to protect the privacy of patients in case of illegal transmission, revision or data loss.
37	Dispute settlement	Parties to the service shall agree on how to settle disputes in accordance with laws of the countries they operate in.
38	Service evaluation and improvement	The service provider shall put in place an evaluation management mechanism on international Chinese medicine telemedicine service and carry out specific evaluations with scientific and workable evaluation plans.
39		Data collected shall be authentic. Evaluation results shall be objective and accurate, of high credibility.
40		The service provider shall formulate corrective measures on existing problems in accordance with the evaluation results and shall work on continuous improvement. All is recorded.